YOUR IMMUNE SYSTEM

Are you taking care of it?

Holly Fourchalk, PhD., DNM®, RHT, HT

CHOICES UNLIMITED
FOR
HEALTH AND WELLNESS

Dr. Holly Fourchalk, Ph.D., DNM®, RHT, HT

Tel: 604.764.5203
Fax: 604.465.7964

Website: www.choicesunlimited.ca
E-mail: holly@choicesunlimited.ca

Interior Design and Cover Design:
Wendy Dewar Hughes, Summer Bay Press
Editing: Julene Schroeder

ISBN: 978-1-927626-36-8
Digital ISBN: 978-1-927626-37-5

This book includes neither an exhaustive nor exclusive list of alternative options for working with the Immune System.

Rather, it provides an overview of theories, foods, herbs and modalities with which the patient or practitioner may work.

My company is called Choices Unlimited for Health and Wellness for a reason. There are lots of choices to choose from with regard to maximizing your health. We can only make good, effective choices when we have a working knowledge of what those choices may be.

If a given modality or protocol resonates for you, research it further. Explore your options within the profile. Your mind is a very powerful tool – make it work for you. Regardless of what you choose to do, make the placebo effect – or the power of the mind – be a part of your healing journey.

Here's to your journey into health.

DISCLAIMER

Every effort has been made by the author to ensure that the information in this book is as accurate as possible. However, it is by no means a complete or exhaustive examination of all information.

The author knows what worked for her and what has worked for others but no two people are the same. Therefore, the author cannot and does not render judgment or advice regarding a particular individual.

Further, because each body is unique, any two individuals may experience different results from the same therapy.

The author believes in both prevention and the superiority of a natural non-invasive approach over drugs and surgery.

The information collected within comes from a variety of researchers and sources from around the world. This information has been accumulated in the western healing arts over the past thirty years.

Research has shown that one of the top three leading causes of death in North America occurs because of the physician/pharmaceutical component of the scenario.

Perhaps the real leading cause of death and disability is a result of the lack of awareness of natural therapies. These therapies are well known to prevent and treat many common degenerative, inflammatory and oxidative diseases.

The author loves to research and loves to teach. This book is another attempt to increase awareness about health and the many options we have to bring the body back into a healthy balance.

Ever-increasing numbers of people are aware of healing foods and herbs, supplements and modalities but there are still far too many who are not. The fact that our physicians are part of this latter group makes healing even more challenging; yet we are now seeing more and more laboratories around the world and more universities in and outside of the U.S. studying herbs, nutrition and various healing modalities with phenomenal success.

The unfortunate fact is that those who can profit from sickness and disease promote ignorance and the results are devastating.

It is not the intent of the author that anyone should choose to read this book and make decisions regarding his or her health or medical care based on ideas contained in this book.

It is the responsibility of the individual to find a health care practitioner to work with to achieve optimal health.

The author and publisher are not responsible for any adverse effects or consequences resulting from the use of any of the suggestions or information contained in the book but offer this material as information that the public has a right to hear and utilize at its own discretion.

To my Parents

For all their support and encouragement
My Dad for his ever-listening ear
My mother for her open mind

CONTENTS

PART ONE

UNDERSTANDING YOUR IMMUNE SYSTEM

ONE

The history of understanding our immune system

"'Tis healthy to be sick sometimes."

Henry David Thoreau

The immune system plays a gigantic part in our overall health and needs to be exercised regularly, just like any muscle. Understanding how it works and how we can support its health is paramount if we want to live a long, healthy, high-quality life.

You will find this book divided into three parts:

Part I—We will explore the immune system, what it does, and its composition.

Part II—We will explore dysfunctions in the immune system and how they impact different parts of the body.

We will also explore what we need to do to maintain a good healthy immune system or to recover when the digestive tract has suffered ill health.

1

The book is organized so that you do not have to read Chapter 1 to understand Chapter 5; rather, you can go directly to the parts that interest you most and then return to the parts that will give you further understanding.

The history of understanding the immune system is very complicated. Each culture developed its own understanding of it. Let's start with the western culture.

Western Civilization

In western medicine, the immune system was first recognized in 430 B.C. when it was noted that people who had already suffered the plague and recovered could nurse the sick without becoming re-infected.

Nothing much happened between then and the 1800s when there were three scientists who were independently exploring similar scientific experiments in chemistry. They were all working with fermentation and bacteria. These three men were Louis Pasteur, Antoine Bechamp, and Robert Koch.

While not working together, they were somewhat aware of what each of the others was doing and were in competition. They apparently lied, stole research and presented fraudulent research in an attempt to gain the opportunity to address royalty, the medical society, or a university.

Unfortunately, Louis Pasteur won the race and established the "Germ Theory." Germ theory states that microorganisms can cause disease, such as:

- Virus: Small infectious agent that replicates itself inside the cells of another organism, such as animals, plants or bacteria.
- Bacterium: A large domain of microorganisms with various shapes which allow for classification and can be identified as spheres, rods and spirals.
- Fungus: A large group of organisms that includes yeasts, moulds and mushrooms.
- Prions: Infectious agents composed of misfolded proteins.
- Protists: A variety of unicellular, microorganisms, which are "animal-like" protozoa, "plant-like" protophyta (algae) or "fungus-like" (slime or water moulds).

Too small to be seen, these pathogens have the capacity to invade and cause problems in a host. Their growth and reproduction cause the disease.

Interestingly, Louis Pasteur instructed his family not to release his notes until after his death. His grandson released them, some 10,000 pages, in 1975. Dr. Geison, from Princeton and a member of the editorial board of the Journal of the History of Medicine (among other positions), studied Pasteur's notes and presented an address to the American Association for the Advance of Science in Boston in 1993.

Dr. Geison claimed that, "Pasteur published much fraudulent data and was guilty of many counts of "scientific misconduct," violating rules of medicine, science, and ethics."[1] According to Dr. Geison's account:

- Pasteur lacked training and credentials in medicine and physiology; he was a chemist.

- Pasteur very likely created the disease known as "hydrophobia," as opposed to actually finding a cure for it. (The American Psychiatric Institute and other programs vote on new diseases regularly.)

- Pasteur initiated the practice of vivisection with horrific animal experiments. Hundreds of thousands of laboratory animals were killed needlessly in the name of science (in the Pasteurian Institutes and in medical research laboratories ever since).

- Pasteur was directly responsible for the deaths of hundreds of people who were inoculated with unproven vaccines and injections (not unlike creating autism or diseases and death with drugs and injections today).

- He indirectly caused thousands more deaths by introducing people to the administration of unproven Pasteurian procedures. It is interesting to note that still over 50% of medical procedures have never been clinically tested today.

- Was he a merchant or a scientist? He frequently reported false test findings and data for the purpose of self-promotion and profiteering from the sale of drugs and vaccines that were often made mandatory by legislators (just as today).

- He is claimed to have treated (and killed) Alexander, the King of Greece, for a disease he did not even have. (Even today, there is an estimated 72% misdiagnosis in emergency rooms, making physicians and prescription drugs the number one killer in North America.)

- Rather than do experiments on those who were already sick, Pasteur injected disease into healthy subjects.

- In a lecture given in London on 25 May 1911, M.L. Leverson, MD stated: "The entire fabric of the germ theory of disease rests upon assumptions which not only *have not been proved*, but which are incapable of proof, and many of them can be proved to be the reverse of truth. The basic one of these unproven assumptions, wholly due to Pasteur, is the hypothesis that all the so-called infectious and contagious disorders are caused by germs"[2] (italics mine.)

Koch, like Pasteur, lied for money and fame. They both received money for their work, despite it not being proven, creating the marriage between health, science and marketing.

Bechamp, the third scientist of that time, a professor and true researcher, discovered tiny organisms called "microzymas," that he claimed were present in animals, plants, and minerals. Bechamp claimed that these organisms would take on different forms depending on the condition of the host. If the host was diseased, these microzymas became pathological viruses and bacteria. Bechamp claimed that it was not the bug that caused the disease but rather the environment that the bugs lived in, i.e. in a low-resistance, weak immune system. His theories have never been refuted, yet they have never made headway in the modern health sciences.

Unfortunately, Pasteur's concepts of Germ Theory did receive recognition and formed the basis of modern western medicine – much to the detriment of patients today. Greed, politics and pharmaceutical economics all took precedence over health.

Now that Pasteur's work has been released, we know that he retracted the Germ Theory on his deathbed. He acknowledged that Bernard had been right and that it was not the germ that caused the problem but rather the environment in which the germ was found.

TCM/Traditional Chinese Medicine

In China, the concept of Germ Theory was quite different. They started where Louis Pasteur left off. TCM believes that a pathogen can only attack or develop if there is weakness in the system. "Germs gather and thrive only in weakened parts of the body of patients with low resistance...Germs simply cannot attack strong healthy organs."[2] To kill the pathogen without healing the underlying weakness simply leaves one susceptible to the pathogen attacking again.

Long before western conventional medicine began to develop, Chinese medical practitioners knew that it was the environment that allowed a pathogen to grow. It was not the pathogen that caused the problem.

Ayurvedic Medicine

In India, it was believed that the cause of disease and dysfunction was the result of imbalances in the body. The Ayurvedic definition of health recognized the connection between the mind and the body *and* that health was more than the absence of disease; it was a dynamic state of balance and integration of body, mind and spirit. They believed if we took care of the body using the following methods we would have better health:

- Ayurvedic massage
- Detoxification protocols
- Herbs
- Diet
- Yoga
- Aromatherapy
- Meditation

Again, this kind of program supports an understanding that when we create health in the body, germs cannot develop. Modern conventional medicine is starting to recognize this age-old truth.

With this brief historical understanding of the theories of health and how western conventional medicine became sidetracked into the allopathic model, let's examine the immune system.

TWO

Your immune system: What is you and what isn't you?

Did you know that your immune system is partly you and partly not you? Consider the following information about our immune system:

- The immune system is made up two primary components:
  - Cells
  - Bacteria that we require.
- About 90% of immune system is in the gut.
- The immune system is the cause of allergies.
- The immune system has a vast number of different components.
- The immune system is tremendously undeveloped at birth and takes about three years to develop fully.
- The first dose of bacteria happens as we travel through the vaginal canal.
- The majority of both the immune system and the bacteria are in the gut.

- We have over a 1000 different types of bacteria in the gut alone.

- These bacteria both support and provoke the immune system.

- The immune system also involves a huge number of specialized cells that we create.

- Many of those immune cells can be programed.

Parts of the immune system

The organs of the immune system are distributed throughout the entire body. The immune system is a diverse system with vessels that parallel the blood/cardiovascular system. It also interacts with and overlaps other systems and thus can be difficult to identify, define and describe. But let's give it a shot.

The immune system can be broken down in two different ways. The first is a general overview. However, if you are more interested in a better understanding of the terms and functions of the immune system, you can find that in Chapter 4.

The following is a brief breakdown that may help you put the immune system into perspective. Notice where the inflammatory system fits into the immune system.

First, very simply, the immune system is composed of **what is us**:

- Organs
- Tissues
- Vessels
- Nodes

Innate immune system

Our innate immunity is responsible for the following:

- First line of defense against infection
- Defense mechanism for responding to pathogens: viruses, bacteria, mould, fungus, etc.
- Brings immune cells to the problem area to identify, respond and eliminate the pathogen or germ
- Provokes the initiation of the complement cascade system that identifies the pathogen
- Triggers inflammatory cells
- Tags pathogens for other cells to kill
- Causes death in pathogens
- Involves different types of white blood cells to remove the pathogen
- NK cells
- Mast cells

- Basophils
- Eosinophils
- Phagocytes
- Macrophages
- Neutrophils
- Dendritic cells
- Provokes the adaptive immune system, if necessary
- Provides a barrier to the chemical or pathogen in order to protect the body
- Includes the inflammatory response mechanism, which is considered a stereotyped response vs. a learned adaptive response (adaptive immune system).

Inflammatory System

Adaptive Immune system

Our adaptive immunity is different than the generalized innate immune system because it is responsible for:

- Highly specific cells
- Systemic cells/processes that eliminate pathogens
- Having a memory of pathogens that have invaded before
- Responding, therefore, stronger each time the pathogen presents itself

- Being a system that learns and is thus adaptive
- Cellular immunity: T cell
- Humoral system (means in fluids): B cells
- Lymph (lymph fluid runs through all the vessels that parallel the cardiovascular system)

For those who are interested, there is a more specific breakdown of the immune system in Chapter 4.

What isn't us:

- Bacterial system
- More than 10,000 microbial species in the human system[1]
- Over 1000 different bacteria in the small and large intestines
- Only four bacterial groups and yeast can survive in the hydrochloric acid of the stomach
- Skin microbiota has over 1000 species from nineteen species/phyla
- Skin and vaginal sites show smaller diversity from person to person
- Urogenital tract has a varied flora depending on age, pH and hormone levels of the host
- Eyelids have a progressive change in flora throughout one's life

- The mouth contains fourteen different phyla of bacteria
- The lower respiratory tract, bronchi and alveoli do not have flora
- There is also a variety of yeasts and other entities.

Until very recently, none of the flora was well studied. Now science is recognizing that all these microbiota do not simply co-exist but play a vital role in our health and in particular to our immune system.

THREE

The individual parts of our immune system

Organs/Tissues/Vessels/Nodes

Although there are different ways to identify and classify the immune system, many think of the immune system as the lymphoid system of organs that contribute to the regulation of:

- Growth
- Development
- Release of lymphocytes

The organs of the **immune/adaptive/lymph** system include:

- Adenoids: Where the nose transitions into the throat.
- Appendix: Where the small intestine moves into the large intestine. It is rich with lymphoid cells but conventional medicine thought it was unnecessary, an old evolutionary structure that had lost its necessity.
- Bone marrow: In the heads of large bones.

17

- Thymus: A lymph structure that is largest in childhood and atrophies in adolescence; can extend from thorax up to thyroid.

- Lymph nodes: Throughout the body but with a high concentration in the armpits and stomach.

- Lymphatic vessels: Vessels that carry lymph to and from the nodes and run parallel to the blood system.

- Peyer's patches: Patches of lymph tissue found in the mucosal membrane in the last stretch of the small intestine and full of lymph cells such as macrophages, dendritic cells, B and T cells.

- Spleen: Organ that is structured like a large lymph node and acts as a blood filter; removes old red blood cells and synthesizes anti-bodies.

- Tonsils: Set of lymphatic tissues found in the throat and includes adenoid tonsil, tubal tonsils and palatine tonsils. Like the thymus, they are largest in childhood and start to atrophy in adulthood. Once again, conventional medicine belief concluded that they were unnecessary even though they form the first major line of defense against pathogens found in the air and food.

Immune cells develop differently. Let's look at some different types.

Immune cells, like all blood cells, begin in the bone marrow, which is the soft tissue in the hollow shafts of long bones. The cells start out as stem cells and become either phagocytes (large white blood cells that ingest microbes, other cells, foreign particles) or lymphocytes (B and T cells).

Immune/Innate

- Phagocytes: Ingest pathogens, harmful foreign particles, dying cells; they are classified as professional (more effective) and non-professional. One litre of human blood contains about six billion phagocytes.
- Monocytes: Replenish macrophages and dendritic cells; they respond to infection and inflammation signals and move fast.
- Macrophage: Clean up dead host cells and non-infectious debris and usually move slowly.
- Neutrophils: Most abundant, about ten produced daily and they last about five and a half days. Neutrophils are a type of macrophage but prefers to ingest simple carbs/sugars rather than bacteria;

fasting strengthens neutrophils; they react in infections and inflammations.

- Dendritic cells: found in skin and other areas that are in direct contact with the environment; have long tentacles/dendrites that capture pathogens; activate T cells

- Mast cells: interact with dendritic cells, B and T cells; help mediate adaptive immune functions; consume and kill some types of bacteria such as salmonella; secrete histamine.

Immune/Adaptive/Lymphocytes:

- B cells manoeuvre through their maturation process in the bone marrow. Development proceeds through the IgM+ stage in the bone. Then they move to the lymphoid tissue (spleen, lymph nodes or Peyer's patches, which are lymph nodes in the small intestine) where they are called transitional B cells. Some graduate into mature B-lymphocytes whereby they are typically identified by a protein on the outer surface, which allows them to bind a specific type of molecule.

- T cells, on the other hand, travel to the thymus for maturation. They have specific types of receptors (CD4 or CD8) that evolve through their development in the thymus. About 2% reach full maturation and then travel to peripheral tissues. The thymus starts to shrink in early childhood and consequently, there is a corresponding drop to the number of T cells.

- The lymphatic system, is a big part of the adaptive immune system, and runs parallel to the circulatory system. It is a system that:
  - o Recycles blood plasma
  - o Removes interstitial fluid
  - o Transports white blood cells between bones and lymph nodes
  - o Absorbs and transports fatty acids and fats from the digestive tract
  - o Transports needed immune cells to a required location
  - o Unfortunately the lymphatic system can also carry carcinogenic cells that bubble off of tumours to different parts of the body (called metastasis) but thankfully lymph nodes in the system can also trap cancer cells.

What isn't us

Microbiota

The microbiota, microflora or microbiome refer to the community of microorganisms that **are not us** but live in us. The majority of these organisms are beneficial to our health. However, if most of them are depleted then there can be a problem. For instance, we can have problems if:

- A and B are not balanced
- C is predominant over D rather than vice versa
- There is an insufficiency of F and G

In addition, there are many microorganisms that are pathogenic, i.e. they disrupt the effective functioning of our bodies. The majority are predominantly bacterial but there are also versus, viral, yeast and mould, etc. There are more than ten times the number of bacterial cells in our gut than human cells in the body. And they play an important role.

Prior to birth, the fetus is basically sterile of any bacteria. The first dose of bacteria comes as the baby struggles through the vaginal canal. (This is one of the many reasons why the World Health Organization [WHO] is so against the high number of caesarians in North America). The baby bacterial profile of the immune system continues to develop in the gut with continued doses of bacteria found in the mother's milk, through the food formulas, and finally through the food.

Of course, during that time the skin also develops a bacterial level through touch. The respiratory develops through breathing.

Let's look at another component of the immune system in the gut. It is called the "gut barrier." The surface of the gut lining, called the "epithelial layer," is also a part of our immune system.

This lining is specialized to perform a number of different functions:

- Protects the body from pathogens
- Absorbs nutrients from the gastrointestinal tract into the body
- Houses many of the immune cells that destroy pathogens trying to move through it into our body

Unfortunately, a number of issues can break down and destroy this barrier:

- A wide number of drugs
- Antibiotics
- Pain killers

- Ant-acids, NSAIDS (Motrin, Advil, Aleve, Vioxx, etc),
- NSAIDS (Motrin, Advil, Aleve, Vioxx, etc.)
- An acidic diet
- Sugar
- Sodas
- Deli Meats, corned beef, salamis, etc.
- Cheeses: low fat cheddar, hard cheese, processed cheese, Parmesan cheese
- Junk Foods
- Fast Foods
- Nutrient deficiency of: amino acids, Omega 3s, anti-oxidants, vitamins and minerals, phytonutrients
- Environmental toxins: persistent organic pesticides, pesticides, insecticides, herbicides:
  o Butylated Hydroxyanisole (BHA) in chewing gum, diaper creams, snack food
  o Bisphenol A (BPA), as in water bottles, baby bottles, plastic wraps, food packaging
  o Oxybenzone, found in sunscreens, lip balm, moisturizers
  o Parabens in moisturizers, hair care and shaving products

- Phthalates in food packaging, shampoo, toys, detergents
- Perfluorooctanioic Acid (PFOA) in non-stick Teflon pans, tap water, perchlorate (an oxidant in rocket fuel that is added to water and soil), vegetables, drinking water
- Decabromodiphenyl Ether (DECA) in materials such as carpets, furniture, electronics
- Asbestos in toys, housing insulation, drywall, artificial fireplace logs[1]
- Heavy metal toxicity: (vegetables take up metals by absorbing them from contaminated soils: "nearly half of the mean ingestion of lead, cadmium and mercury through food is due to plant origin (fruit, vegetables and cereals)."[2]

- **Mercury:**
  - Tooth fillings
  - Water
  - Fish

- **Arsenic:**
  - Chicken
  - Fish
  - Meat

- Rice
- Water
- **Lead:**
  - Plants absorption can exceed several hundred times the maximum levels safe for humans [4]
- **Aluminum:**
  - Cookware
  - Aluminum cans for beer and soft drinks
- **Antacids** (Maalox, Mylants, Gaviscon, Riopan, Alka-seltzer, Rolaids):
  - Hemodialysis
  - Anti-perspirants
  - Baking powder
  - Cosmetics
  - Municipal water supplies
  - Drying agents to keep products dry like: salt, cocoa
  - Emulsifier: processed cheese, flour[5]
- **Zinc:**
  - Vegetables: celery, Chinese cabbage
  - Oysters
  - Red meat
  - Seafood: crab and lobster
  - Whole grains, fortified breakfast cereals

- Dairy products
- Phylates which attach to zinc in various foods attach and prevent its absorption
- Whole grain breads, cereals, legumes[6]
- **Copper:** Zinc and manganese deficiencies which cause copper retention in:
    - Water lines
    - Vegetables
    - Meats and eggs
    - Nuts and seeds
    - Grains
    - Multi vitamin
- **Water supplies:**
    - Arsenic
    - Barium
    - Cadmium
    - Chromium
    - Copper
    - Lead
    - Mercury
    - Nickel
    - Selenium
    - Thallium [7]

Chronic stress: All of the above can disrupt the:

- Gut
- Gut lining
- Inflammatory system in the gut and elsewhere
- Immune system in the gut and elsewhere
- Microbiota in the gut and elsewhere

Whether these issues are transferred from the mother, absorbed through the diet, or absorbed through water and drugs, they can have a huge impact on our system and we need either to prevent them or take care of them.

FOUR

A more in-depth look at the immune system

I promised a more extensive breakdown of the immune system for those who were interested.

Innate: first line of defense that is made up of:

- Complement system:
    - Made up of over 20 different proteins that work as antibodies
    - Triggers the inflammatory system
    - Leukocytes: white blood cells
    - Approximately 7000 white blood cells/1 microliter of blood

The following is a simple chart of different types of immune cells and what they stem from:

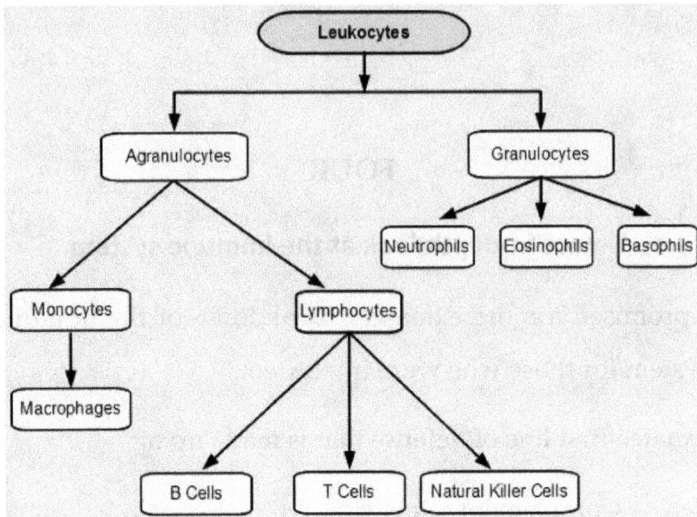

- Natural killer cells (destroy compromised cells like tumour cells or virus-infected cells)
  - o Mast cells: found in connective tissues and mucous membranes; regulate the inflammatory response; and release histamine, a vasodilator, in the allergic response
  - o Eosinophils: secrete chemicals in response to parasites and various infections
  - o Basophils: similar to the mast cell, secrete histamine, respond in inflammatory situations forming an anticoagulant - heparin - that prevents blood from clotting too quickly

30

- Phagocytic cells:
  - Phagocytes: eat or engulf pathogens or compounds that should not be there
  - Phagosomes/lysosomes
  - Macrophages: found in tissues and produce a variety of chemicals and enzymes, complement proteins and regulatory factors; but they are also scavengers
  - Neutrophils: 50-60% of phagocytes, found predominantly in the in the blood; target bacteria and fungi
  - Dendritic cells: found in tissues that interact with the external environment, i.e. nose, gastro-intestinal tract
- Inflammatory system
  - Eicosanoids: signalling molecules made from Omega 3 and 6 fatty acids
  - Prostaglandins: produce fever, dilation of blood vessels
  - Leukotrienes: attract the Leukocytes above
  - Cytokines: signal molecules made from proteins

31

- Interleukins: communicate between white blood cells
- Chemokines: provoke chemotaxis or movement
- Interferons: anti-viral effects

Adaptive: This is the part of the immune system that has memory and thus evolves, which is why it is called adaptive or acquired. The adaptive response is antigen- or pathogen-specific as opposed to the generalized reaction of the innate system.

- Lymphocytes: we have about two trillion lymphocytes and these make up between 20-40% of the white blood cells
- B cells: involved in the humoral response system noted above. Each B cell recognizes a different type of pathogen. They have specific types of receptors on the cell surface that binds to different types of antigen or pathogen. When an antigen is detected, the B cell secretes a free form of those receptors, which are now antibodies; the antibodies break down the antigen using proteolysis (breaks up the proteins). There are five classes of antibodies:

- IgA: antibodies that play a role in mucosal linings (about 3-5 gms are secreted into the intestinal lining every day)
- IgA1: found in mucosal linings and in the blood
- IgA2: found in body secretions

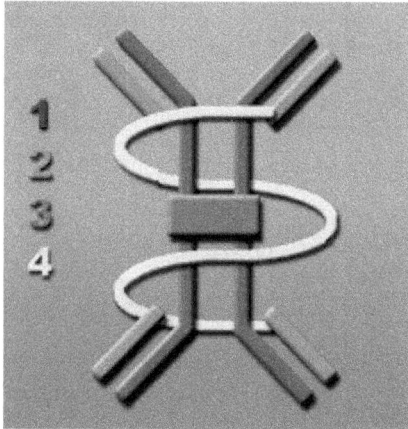

- IgD: activates B cells; binds to basophils and mast cells to activate them as well
- IgE: responds to parasitic worms and allergies like asthma and anaphylactic reactions

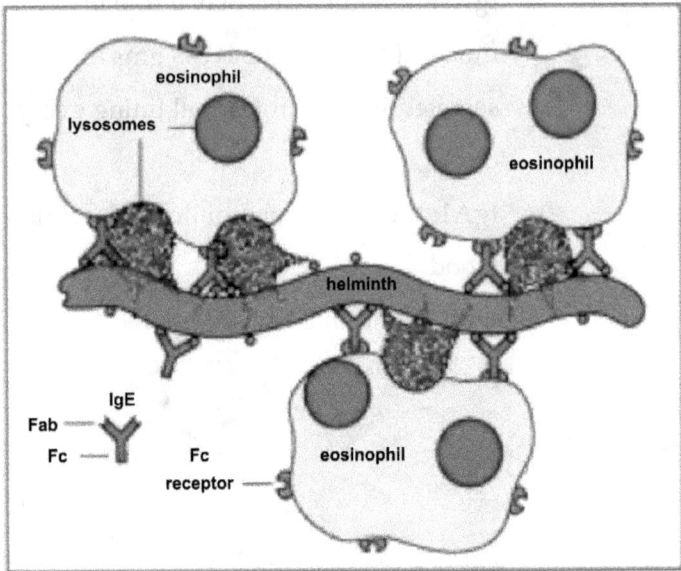

IgG: binds to pathogens in the blood and extracellular fluids like bacteria, viruses and fungi, making them identifiable to the phagocytes that ingest them.

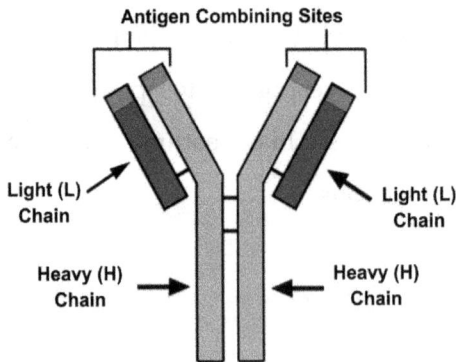

- o IgM: an antibody produced by B cells in the spleen

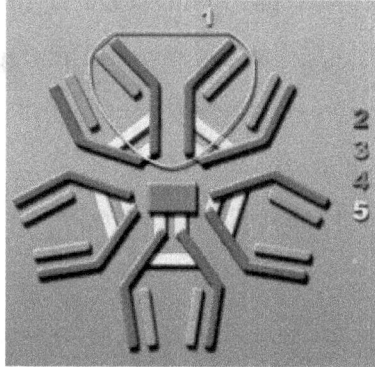

- T cells: involved in cell mediated responses – connects with a tagged cell and release cell toxins or cytotoxins into the cell, causing cell death or apoptosis
- Killer T cells: recognize one type of pathogens that have already been tagged by a Class 1 MHC; cells that have already been infected or are otherwise damaged/ dysfunctional and cause cell death with cytotoxins
- Helper T cells: recognize a differ type of pathogen that has been tagged by the Class 11 MHC; also regulate the innate and adaptive responses and release communicator molecules called cytokines

- T-helper 1: Th1 – produce interferon – that coats the pathogen and gamma that activates the B cells to respond (used when a cell is infected)
- T-helper 2: Th2 – release Interleukin 4 – which also trigger activation of B cells (used with a pathogen outside of the cell)
- Natural killer T cells: straddle both sides of the innate and adaptive systems

FIVE

The inflammatory component of the immune system

As we noted previously, the inflammatory system is part of the immune system. Like different parts of the immune system and different components in our body, the inflammatory system operates in different systems when required.

If there is trauma to a bone, muscle, organ, etc., the inflammatory system will kick in. In fact, even when you are lying on your bed, just breathing, you can have breakage in your arterioles (the smallest of the arteries) which causes an inflammatory response. On the other hand, it also operates as part of the immune system, protecting you from pathogens.

So let's review what part the inflammatory system plays in the immune system.

The inflammatory system is part of the innate–humoral system in the body. "Innate" means that it does not have to be trained like the cells in the adaptive system and "humoral" means that it is found in the body fluids.

37

The particular compounds found in the inflammatory component of the immune system are:

- Eicosanoids: signal molecules made from Omega 3 and six fatty acids
- Cytokines: signal molecules made from proteins
- Prostaglandins: produce fever, dilate blood vessels
- Leukotrienes: attract the Leukocytes/white blood cells (natural killer cells, mast cells, eosinophils, basophils)
- Interleukins: communicate between white blood cells
- Chemokines: provoke chemotaxis or movement
- Interferons: anti-viral effects
- Macrophages: engulf and digest cellular by-products and pathogens
- Dendritic cells: provide communication between cells using proteins or interferon and cytokines
- Histiocytes: macrophages found in tissues
- Kupffer cells: a specialized macrophage in the lining of the liver
- Mastocytes: or a mast cell, well known for releasing histamine in allergic reactions, but also very important in wound healing

Once the inflammatory system has begun its process of creating permeability in the blood vessels, we have leakage. This leakage is called exudation. The exudation or leakage of proteins (fibrin proteins for clotting and immunoglobulins which are antibodies) and fluids into the surrounding area causes the swelling.

Once the exudation process begins, other systems are provoked:

- Vascular system: changes in the blood system that increase the size and permeability of the blood vessels, thus allowing necessary molecules to move wherever needed
- Plasma blood system: which is comprised of the complement system, the kinin system, the coagulation system and the fibrinolysis system.
- Complement system: part of the immune system that promotes:
  o Opsonisation: process of tagging pathogens. This will be activated even if the inflammation is a result of a broken bone or physical trauma to the body. An injured site is a great place for pathogens already in the body to create a new home. If the injured site opens the body to the outside, then

pathogens, which were not part of the body previously, may find a new home. The body needs to be prepared for this possibility.

- o Chemotaxis: is about movement – both our body compounds and pathogens will make movement to the injured area in response to signalling compounds and other forms of information. For example, hormones are the signalling molecules of the endocrine system, neurotransmitters signal for the nervous system, and cytokines signal for the immune system.
- o Agglutination: the process whereby either red blood cells or white blood cells bind together
- o Produces MAC: this membrane-attack complex forms on the surface of a pathogen leading to death

- Kinin System: this system, although poorly understood, involves large blood proteins and some enzymes that activate and deactivate different compounds. Some of the components are vasodilators. The system plays a role in:
  - o Inflammation
  - o Blood pressure
  - o Coagulation

- Pain (Bradykinin)
- Coagulation System: the process by which blood forms clots. When a blood vessel wall is damaged, the coagulation system covers the wall with a platelet and fibrinogen to stop the bleeding and begin the repair work with clotting factors.
- Fibrinolysis System: this system prevents the coagulation system from getting out of control. It has two components: the first part is the normal regulatory system that prevents blood clots from continuing to grow; the second part occurs in reaction to pharmaceutical drugs or a medical disorder.

Then the cellular system gets involved. This system involves the leukocytes, which are found in the blood and need to move to the injured area.

- Leukocytes: There are a number of different types of leukocytes that are involved in both the initiation and process of inflammation:
  - Leukocytes need to be signalled
  - Leukocytes then need to travel
  - Leukocytes then need to do their work
- Cell mediators: some of the cell mediators include:

41

- o Nitric oxide: relaxes the smooth muscles of the arteries allowing for vasodilation to occur
- o Prostaglandins: involved in vasodilation as well but also involved in the fever and pain processes
- o Lysosome granules: contain a wide variety of enzymes that are able to break down different substances and others that act as inflammatory mediators
- o Histamine: causes the arteries to dilate and increases permeability in the veins

As you can see, there are a lot of interconnections between the immune system and the inflammatory system. For optimal health to occur, we need both systems and the interconnections between the systems to be working effectively.

Whether the initial disruptions began in the immune system or in the inflammatory system, they often need to communicate for effective resolution of the inflammation and effective elimination of the pathogen.

Having said that, not all pathogens need to be eliminated totally. As long as our immune system has the upper hand and can keep the pathogens under control, we will experience physiological health.

In fact, the presence of pathogens in the system keeps the immune system active and strong, similar to muscles that need occasional workouts to stay strong. The difference is that we don't always need the muscles to be active, but we do want the immune system always to be active and very alert.

PART TWO

THE IMMUNE SYSTEM AND DISEASE

SIX

What happens when the immune system goes out of balance?

As noted, our immune system needs to be working continually. Whether we are awake or asleep, it keeps going, just like our heart. It needs to be nourished with nutrients that allow it to keep producing all the molecules, compounds and cells required to keep going.

When we have an unhealthy diet, when we allow toxins (from our air, food, water, hygiene and cleaning products) to bog down our system, our immune system becomes challenged.

When the immune system is out of balance, it can result in:

- Autoimmune disorders
- Chronic Inflammation

Autoimmune disorders

These disorders are an abnormal response of the immune

system and/or the inflammatory system to the body. Due to a dysfunction, the immune system now perceives aspects of the natural functioning body to be the enemy. The part of the body, which is under attack, may be an organ, such as autoimmune thyroiditis, or it may be a type of tissue.

Typically these disorders arise because the adaptive or innate immune systems went awry. There are more than 80 recognized autoimmune disorders that may be chronic or debilitating, through to fatal. The immune system responds to a pathogen, which is the antigen, and may be a:

- Bacteria
- Virus
- Toxin
- Cancer

The body then produces antibodies that destroy the invading antigen but when an autoimmune disorder develops, the body mistakes some part of the body as the antigen.

When the immune system goes awry, it is in response to a given protein. When the inflammatory system goes awry, it is typically an overreaction of signalling factors, such as IFN (interferon gamma) or TNF (tumour necrosis factor).

What causes the misunderstanding is largely hypothetical at this point. We do know that drugs can cause autoimmune disorders. But some of the body's own mechanisms may also cause it.

The result of an autoimmune dysfunction may result in:

- Abnormal growth of an organ
- Abnormal function of an organ
- Destruction of an organ or a tissue

Tissues and organs usually affected are:

- Basement membrane: layer of fibres that line the cavities/surfaces of various organs
- Blood vessels: arteries and veins
- Connective tissues: tendon, ligament, muscle, bone
- Endocrine glands: pancreas or thyroid
- Gut: lining of the small and large intestine
- Joints: knees, hands
- Lymphatic organs: spleen, thymus
- Muscles
- Red blood cells
- Skin

With conventional medicine, these autoimmune disorders are treated by suppressing the immune system, which can leave the individual wide open to other infections and dysfunctions. Never mind the fact that synthetic medications deplete nutrients in the body or the fact that medications almost always have side effects.

Alternative medicine attempts to bring the immune system back into balance. One way of doing this can be to work with glutathione. Glutathione is recognized as a basic requirement in all the immune cells. Without glutathione, the immune cells are not capable of developing, maintaining or responding. Glutathione is also utilized in keeping the balance required between different types of immune cells, T1 and T2 cells. If either one becomes dominant, different diseases or dysfunctions will develop.

Another way to bring the immune system back into balance is to work with transfer factor. The initial transfer factors come through the mother during fetal development. When the infant is breast -feeding, the mother's milk provides more antibodies and transfer factors. The transfer factor will in effect retrain the immune system in the gut and bring it back into balance.

Transfer Factor:

- Has the ability to re-program T cell lymphocytes and does it quickly
- Enhances and strengthens the immune system capacity to deal with:
  - Bacterial
  - Fungal
  - Mycobacterial
  - Parasitic
  - Viral
- Regulates an overactive immune system (as in autoimmune disorders) and brings it back into balance.[1]
- Often, even when the issues are not in the gut (because the majority of the immune system resides in the gut), transfer factor will have a broad spectrum impact.

- In addition, the microbiota impact on the immune system but provoking the activity of different types of immune cells.
- Together, the immune system and the microbiota can impact various different areas of the body through different systems like the:
  - Vagus Nerve

49

- Provocation of immune cells
- Epithelial lining of the gut

SEVEN

Weight gain, the gut and the immune system

We all know that obesity is accelerating out of control and is becoming a serious problem for younger and younger children.

We have all heard stats on how sick our population is and how poor our diet is.

Aspects of an unhealthy diet under attack include:

- Way too much sugar
- Way too many sodas
- Way too much GMOs
- Way too many bad fats
- Lack of Omega 3
- Heavy metal toxicity
- Environmental toxicity
- AGEs (Advanced Glycation End products)
- Microwaved foods denaturing the nutrients
- Processed foods lacking nutrients
- Pasteurized foods eliminating nutrients

51

- GMOs (genetically modified organisms) that lack nutrients
- Junk foods
- Fast foods
- Artificial foods

We know that junk food puts on weight and clogs up arteries. But it also has a major effect on the immune system.

Let's go back to the microbiota in our gut that we talked of earlier. When we lose the "good" microbiota the "bad" microbiota can set up house.

Some studies are suggesting that we have about 5% of the microbiota that we should have and that the "bad guys" can cause obesity.

There is evidence indicating the gut microbiota can extract calories from ingested foods and are stored in the host fat cells for later use.[1]

You mean my body is storing calories in my fat cells for its future use? Yes!

Let's take this a step further. Scientists looked at two groups of mice. One group of mice had a 40% higher ratio of body fat, even though they were fed less than their counterparts. They took the gut microbiota from the first group and transplanted it into a second group of mice. The second group of mice increased their body weight by 60% in two weeks with no difference in food consumption or energy expenditure/exercise! But there was a 60% increase in weight!

The second group of mice not only had an increase in body fat but, in addition, they:

- Developed insulin resistance
- Had adipocyte hypertrophy (excess body fat)
- Had increased levels of blood glucose
- Developed increased levels of circulating leptin (a hormone that stimulates the sense of hunger and a variety of other issues).[5]

All because their gut bacteria was changed!

Does this mean we can take probiotics and eat junk and lose weight? No. It would appear that the type of microbiota that are able to multiply the best are the ones that like to feed off the food you choose to eat. So if you eat good fats and good fibre, you support the good bacteria. If you eat sugars, artificial food and bad fats, you set up smorgasbord for the "bad guys" to feast on.

Bad Food—Bad Bacteria

Good Food—Good Bacteria

EIGHT

Your immune system and your gut

What happens when your immune system goes astray in your gut? There are a number of gut issues that can arise from either the immune system and/or the inflammatory system.

When we are dealing with inflammatory bowel issues like IBD (usually considered to be autoimmune diseases):

- UC (ulcerative colitis) affects the mucosal lining of the gut
- Crohn's disease can affect any part of the gut
- Collagenous colitis affects the colon
- Lymphocytic colitis causes chronic non-bloody watery diarrhea
- Ischaemic colitis (inflammation/injury) results from inadequate blood supply
- Diversion colitis (inflammation condition as a result of surgery) develops
- Beheet's disease, an immune disorder that affects the mucous membrane, can occur
- Indeterminate colitis

55

Another problem is immune disorders like celiac disease. Celiac patients have ten times the rate of auto-immune thyroid diseases, such as Hashimoto's thyroiditis and Grave's disease, as non-celiac individuals.

NINE

Your immune system and thyroid disease

Hashimoto's thyroiditis is an autoimmune disease that impacts on the thyroid. While there are different theories on what causes hyper thyroid activity, i.e., excessive dietary iodine, one of the evolving theories is that a viral infection may be the cause.

Several studies are suggesting that the gut microbiota may play a big role in Hashimoto's.

We already know that the liver and the adrenals tremendously impact the thyroid, but now we know that the gut also has a huge impact. In fact, the microbiota in the gut are responsible for about 20% of the conversion from T4 to T3! Now we know that the microbiota are very interactive with the immune system in the gut...

Toxicity, in our foods, can also cause thyroid disorders. For instance, bromines are endocrine disruptors. Other chemicals in the same chemical family like fluorine and chlorine, found in our water and food, also cause endocrine disruption because they compete for the iodine receptors on the thyroid.

In addition, these chemicals, along with pesticides; dough conditioners like potassium bromate; brominated vegetable oils; sodium bromates used as emulsifiers, can all harm the immune system in the gut and the microbiota.

When the microbiota is depleted or harmed and/or when the immune system in the gut is harmed, when the gut is inflamed or leaky, the thyroid can be affected.

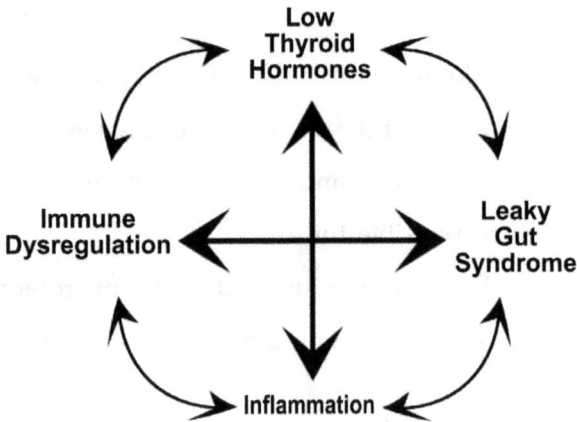

In addition to the gut impacting on the T3 - T4 conversion - the T3 and T4 are required by the gut to keep the gut membrane strong. So there is a strong circular connection between the thyroid, immune system, and the gut microbiota.

TEN

Your immune system, your gut and your brain

Did you know that you have a gut-brain axis that is directional in its communication?

Did you know that it looks like the term "gut-brain axis" is being thrown out in favour of the "microbiota-gut-brain axis"?

"Oh no," you might say, "not back to the gut and the bacteria again!" Yes. Remember, there is ten times more bacteria in your gut than cells in your whole body and 90% of your immune system is in the gut, so yes, we have to keep coming back to the gut and its bacteria.

In my book, *Depression: the real cause may be in your body,* we explored a wide number of physiological issues that can cause depression. Some of those conditions included:

- Acidic pH of the gut
- Deficiency in the gut enzymes
- Deficiency in the microbiota
- The wrong bacteria dominant in the gut
- Leaky gut syndrome

Leaky Gut Syndrome

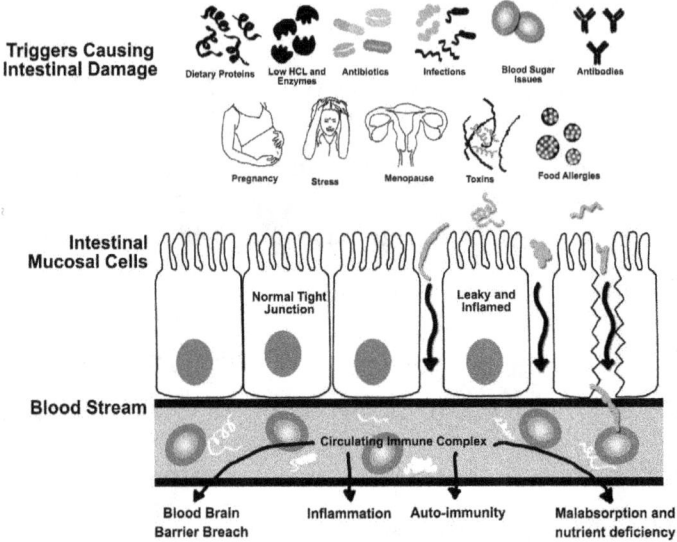

Triggers Causing Intestinal Damage

Dietary Proteins Low HCL and Enzymes Antibiotics Infections Blood Sugar Issues Antibodies

Pregnancy Stress Menopause Toxins Food Allergies

Intestinal Mucosal Cells

Normal Tight Junction

Leaky and Inflamed

Blood Stream

Circulating Immune Complex

Blood Brain Barrier Breach   Inflammation   Auto-immunity   Malabsorption and nutrient deficiency

The typical MDs, psychologists, or psychiatrists, unfortunately, are not assessing these issues. However, they are potent. One of the many reasons I stopped practicing as just a Registered Psychologist in favour of working with the whole body-mind continuum was my discovery of all the physiological conditions that impacted the mind. It is ineffective simply to provide therapy for the mind without understanding all the physiological conditions that can have an impact on the mind or may be major contributing factors.

62

Issues with the gut are only one of several issues that can cause depression. The gut /immune system / microbiota are very intertwined:

- The gut needs to have different pH levels throughout
- The gut requires given nutrients to support the microbiota
- The immune system is mutually dependent on the gut and the microbiota
- The microbiota thrives in a healthy gut
- The immune system is strong when the gut and microbiota are healthy
- A healthy microbiota can trigger the immune system to respond
- A healthy microbiota can take care of given issues such as bad bacteria, which then allow the immune system to focus on other things
- If the gut is toxic, lesioned, leaky or inflamed, the microbiota have a more difficult time functioning.

But how does all of this connect with the brain?

Let's take a short history walk. The first western science recognitions of the gut-brain axis occurred in the 1830s. It was noted that there was a correlation between changing moods and gastric secretions. The belief held until recently was that the information which travelled on this axis was a one way, top-down information line. What we are now learning is that the information is bi-directional and that the gut can have a tremendous impact on the brain, emotions, thoughts and behaviours. Further, it isn't just our gut that is communicating, but rather the microbiota in the gut.

It appears that the gut microbiota communicates with the central nervous system through neural (vagus nerve), endocrine (hormonal) and immune pathways. Thus, the microbiota can impact both brain function and behaviour.[1]

For instance, research shows that there is a direct relationship between the microbiota and the hypothalamic-pituitary adrenal axis.[2]

From early development to old age the gut microbiota impacts the brain. Therefore, the gut microbiota are extremely important to healthy brain development.[3]

The microbiota can influence the development of brain regions involved in how we respond to stress and emotions like anxiety and depression.[4]

Research is showing that the microbiota can impact the brain through the vagus nerve, the tenth cranial nerve that stimulates the gut. Current research also reveals that there is greater activation of the hypothalamus when mice are fed probiotics.[4]

Subsequent studies also show that the microbiota not only impact the brain through the tenth cranial nerve but through the immune system as well. For instance, when mice were infected with Trichuris muris, they had increased inflammation and anxiety. Along the same line, treatment with the probiotic Bifidobacterium longum alleviated anxiety.[5]

The Michael J Fox Foundation is doing a study on the changes in the microbiota associated with Parkinson's Disease.[6]

A press release from Gut Microbiota for Health claims: "FMT (fecal microbiota transplantation) has also been used successfully to treat inflammatory bowel disease, irritable bowel syndrome, obesity and chronic constipation, Parkinson's, chronic fatigue syndrome and autism, FMT has shown to be helpful. The fact that this broad range includes neurological disorders lends additional support to the claim that brain, gut and microbiota are closely connected through an axis formed by a multitude of interrelated paths." [7,8]

ELEVEN

Melatonin and your gut and your immune system

Melatonin is a hormone that historically was believed to be produced and stored only by the pineal gland. It was thought to regulate sleep and circadian rhythms. But that has changed.

Melatonin is now recognized to exhibit a wide spectrum of activities and is produced in various areas of the body, in particular, in the upper portion of the gastrointestinal tract. High concentrations of melatonin are produced in the duodenal unit, which includes the liver, biliary routes and pancreas, in addition to the upper portion of the small intestine. Further, there is much more melatonin made there than in the pineal gland.

Research indicates that the melatonin that is made in the upper GIT location is released into the portal blood flow, where all the other nutrients exit the gastrointestinal tract and enter our bodies. The portal blood then takes melatonin and the other nutrients to the liver where they are further metabolized.[1]

Not only have we found that melatonin is made in various parts of the body but that it is involved in many more activities than previously known. For instance research suggests that melatonin is involved in:

- Circadian movements
- Anti-oxidant properties
- Anti-inflammatory properties
- Anti-cancer benefits:
    o Inhibits a wide range of cancer cell types
    o Prevents tumours from increasing new blood growth, i.e. angiogenesis
    o Decreases toxicity of chemotherapy
    o Counteracts estrogen's ability to stimulate cell growth in cancer cells
    o May stop brain cancers
    o Has been shown to reduce the growth of pancreatic cancer
- Protecting the mucosa lining
- Is now being clinically studied in regards to over 100 different diseases
- Heals gastro-intestinal lesions such as stomatitis, esophagitis, gastritis, and peptic ulcers.[2]

- As the research into the various functions of melatonin expanded, it was recognized that melatonin played a part in the immune system by:
  - Regulating cytokine production (interleukins and tumour necrosis factor). Cytokines are signalling molecules of the immune system.
  - In addition, research suggests that melatonin may also be involved in the production of T cells, a huge component of the adaptive immune system.
  - Stimulates interleukin 2 – another immune cell that helps to identify and attack cells with disordered DNA that may become cancerous.
  - Lack of melatonin will also atrophy your thymus gland which is part of your immune system.
  - Preventing adhesion molecules from "sticking" Leukocytes to the endothelial cells (these are the cells that line the blood vessels, the lymphatic vessels, the gastro-intestinal tract, etc.).[3]

So what can we make of this? If you are having issues with your sleep, it may be the result of your stomach not producing enough melatonin.

If you are having issues with infections or gastro inflammation and other gut issues, it may be the result of not producing enough melatonin in the gut.

But should you just simply take melatonin? No. Melatonin is a hormone and, like any other hormone, it comes with risks:

- Your body is less likely to make something itself if you keep supplementing it.
- Frequent use of melatonin can trigger vicious cycles in the brain.

Now that we know melatonin is utilized for all these different functions and probably many that haven't been discovered yet, we may be throwing off even more natural processes.

Ways to improve natural melatonin production:

- Don't read, text or watch TV in bed. Go to sleep.
- Use less artificial lighting. Go to sleep when it is dark, get up when it is light. While we may not always live by this, especially in the North, it is a good reminder.
    - Light talks to the suprachiasmatic part of the brain (hypothalamus) through the eyes, which talk to the pineal gland and tell it when to release melatonin.
    - Rather than using white and blue lights, use yellow, orange or red lights in the evening.

- Get lots of good sunlight, especially early morning sun.

- Take a good warm bath / shower ninety minutes before bedtime. For even better results, end with a quick dose of cold water.

As with any other medication, natural or synthetic, take melatonin judiciously, with responsibility and awareness.

TWELVE

How to create a healthy gut/immune/ inflammatory system

A gluten free diet

A gluten free diet will decrease the number of firmicutes and increase the number of proteobacteria. This will help to create a good balance in the microbiota. In addition, it has been shown that an increase of Lactobacillus casei can have an impact on the lymph integrity with mice that have celiac.

Diet chelators

One of the problems that can disrupt our immune system and play havoc with our microbiota is heavy metal toxicity. If we have a problem with heavy metal toxicity there are a number of foods we can include in our diet to help detox our bodies of these metals:

- Pectin: found in the rinds of fruits and vegetables:
  - Lemons
  - Cabbage
  - Granny Smith apples
  - Beets
  - Carrots

- Cilantro/Coriander great for:
  - Mercury
  - Aluminum
  - Lead

  and can cross the blood/brain barrier to protect the brain

- Cruciferous vegetables: (increase detoxifying enzymes)
  - Broccoli
  - Kale
  - Cabbage
- Amino acids:
  - Eggs
  - Fish
- Alpha Lipoic Acid
  - Broccoli
  - Brussels sprouts
  - Peas
  - Spinach
- Chlorella and parsley are mild chelators[1]

Diet	Bacteria Altered	Effect on Bacteria
High-fat	*Bifidobactera* spp. (Good)	Decreased (absent)
High-fat and high-sugar	*Clostridium innocuum, Catenbacterium mitsuokai and Enterococcus* spp. (Bad)	Increased
	Bacteriodes spp. (Good)	Decreased
Carbohydrate-reduced	Bacteroidetes (Good)	Increased
Calorie-restricted	*Clostridium cocoides, Lactobacillus* spp. and *Bifidobactera* spp. (Good)	Decreased (growth prevented)
Complex Carbohydrates	*Mycobacterium avium* subspeacies *paratuberculosis* and *Enterobacteriaceae* (Bad)	Decreased
	B. longum subspecies *longum,* *B. breve* and *B. thetaiotaomicron* (Good)	Increased
Refined Sugars	*C. difficile* and *C. Perfringens* (Bad)	Increased
Vegetarian	*E. Coli* (Bad)	Decreased
High *n*-6 PUFA from safflower oil	Bacteroidetes (Good)	Decreased

	Firmicutes, Actinobacteria and Proteobacteria (Good)	Increased
	δ-*Proteobacteria* (Bad)	Increased
Animal Milk Fat	δ-*Proteobacteria* (Bad)	Increased

2

Probiotics

If the gut microbiota is out of balance, why not simply take probiotics to bring the balance back? The problem is that we have 100 trillion bacteria in the gut so taking small doses of probiotics will take a long time to have an impact.

In addition, most probiotic supplements drop the probiotics off in the duodenum, the beginning of the small intestine, whereas we need them at the end of and throughout the large intestine.

Some recommend that if you want to rebalance the gut microbiota you need to take 20-40 billion bacteria per dose as a minimum.[3]

Glutathione

Glutathione is a hugely important compound in the body. It is involved in so many processes in the body. In a healthy body, glutathione is made in every cell of the body. When it comes to the Immune System, glutathione plays a really important part, it is required for the immune system to develop, maintain and respond. It is always required to regulate the balances between different types of immune cells, i.e. Th1 and Th2.

Unfortunately, we cannot just take glutathione as a supplement. The compound will break down in the gut and we lose important components. Even if it stays together, it is too large to cross over any cell membrane. So we need to enable the body's capacity to make glutathione.

Often the body is not making glutathione because it does not have the nutrients to make glutathione. But just as often, it is because the DNA is turned off and the body cannot make the tools that make the glutathione.

So we have products that can turn on the DNA, in order to make the mRNA tools that make the glutathione. We also have a various different formulas that provide the nutrients to make the different types of glutathione. Unfortunately, many of them only provide the nutrients for one time of glutathione without recognition that there are 8 different glutathione compounds in the body.

With the DNA turned on, the mRNA tools created and sufficient glutathione made in the body, our immune system will be able to continue to develop, maintain and respond effectively.

Transfer Factor

Transfer factor is another ingredient important to the glutathione. There are 8 different types of transfer factor found in the body and 6 are found in the gut. Transfer factor was so named because it "transfers" the immune profile from the mother to the newborn. But even as adults, when the immune system is out of balance or distorted, transfer factor can help restore the system.

Transfer factor is found in the colostrum of mother's milk of any mammal. Scientists have researched transfer factor around the world. Like other supplements it is important to take the authentic compound and not a synthetic version of it.

Like with glutathione, transfer factor can have a huge impact on the immune system in the gut and throughout the body.

THIRTEEN

Concluding remarks

We started out by saying: The immune system plays a gigantic part in our overall health and needs to be exercised regularly, just like any muscle. Understanding how it works and how we can support its health is paramount if we want to live a long, healthy, high-quality life.

Throughout this book, we have explored how the immune system plays a huge part, not only in defending us against pathogens and pathogenic microbes but also how the interaction between the immune system and the microbiota in the gut help different parts of the body to function effectively, i.e. convert T3 to T4.

A common current recognition is that *inflammation* is the *"Silent Killer"*. We also know that the Inflammatory System is part of the Immune System. Many claim that inflammation is the most common cause of disease and dysfunction in today's world. But true exploration requires us to look at what is causing the inflammation and/or the immune system to go out of balance.

We now know that there are a wide range of issues that can cause imbalances, dysfunctions and distortions in the immune system, which we can categorize in the following manner:

- Heavy metal toxicity & other toxicities
- Nutrient deficiency
- Imbalance in the microbiota
- Other organ dysfunction

We also now know, how we can:

- Clean up the body
- Restore the nutrients
- Restore the microbiota
- Help restore other organ dysfunction

The choice is yours. Do you take a few steps in the present to protect your health in the long run. OR ... Are you willing to put your health on the back burner and suffer down the road.

Here's to good choices and long-term health.

References and Quotes

ONE

[1] O'shea, Tim. The Post-Anti-biotic Age: Germ Theory. Found in: http://www.whale.to/vaccine/shea1.html

[2] Ibid

[3] Different theory between Western Medicine and Traditional Chinese Medicine in the causes of disease. Found in:
http://www.chineseherbal.com.au/western_medicine_tcm.htm

TWO

[1] http://en.wikipedia.org/wiki/Human_Microbiome_Project

THREE

[1] Environmental Toxins. Found in:
http://content.time.com/time/specials/packages/article/0,28804,1976909_1976895_1976903,00.html

[2] Islam, Ejaz ul, et al. Assessing potential dietary toxicity of heavy metals in selected vegtables and food crops. Found in:
http://www.ncbi.nlm.nih.gov/pmc/articles/PMC1764924/

[3] Arsenic Poisoning Found In:

http://www.medindia.net/patients/patientinfo/arsenic
-poisoning.htm#·

[4] Wierzbicka M. How lead loses its toxicity to plants. Acta Soc Bot Pol. 1995;64:81–90

[5] Aluminum Toxicity. Found in:
http://www.arltma.com/Articles/AlumToxDoc.htm

[6] Office of Dietary Supplements: Zinc Found In:
http://ods.od.nih.gov/factsheets/Zinc-
HealthProfessional/

[7] Metals in DrinkingWater. Found In:
http://extoxnet.orst.edu/faqs/safedrink/metals.htm

SIX

[1] Bennett, Richard, Ph.D. Inflammation, Health and Longevity. Red Point Publishers, Utah. 2006.

TEN

[1] Cryan, JF, TG Dinan. Mind-altering microorganisms: the impact of the gut microbiota on brain and behaviour. Found In:

http://www.ncbi.nlm.nih.gov/pubmed/22968153

[2] Dinan, TG, JF Cryan. Regulation of the stress response by the gut microbiota: implications for psychoneuroendocrinology. Found In:

http://www.ncbi.nlm.nih.gov/pubmed/22483040

[3] Lyte, M., Li, W., Opitz, N., Gaykema, R.P., and Goehler, L.E. (2006). Induction of anxiety-like behavior in mice during the initial stages of infection with the agent of murine colonic hyperplasia Citrobacter rodentium. Physiol Behav 89, 350-357.

[4] Foster, Jane. Gut Feelings: Bacteria and ther Brain. Found in:

http://dana.org/news/cerebrum/detail.aspx?id=44080

[5] https://www.michaeljfox.org/foundation/grant-detail.php?grant_id=933

[6] Arnous, Pierre-Yves. Press Release – Faecal microbiota transplantation cures gastrointestinal diseases. Found in:

http://www.gutmicrobiotaforhealth.com/t/thu-26-pr-gmfh-87

ELEVEN

[1] Konturek, SJ, et al. Localization and biological activities of melatonin in intact and diseased gastrointestinal tract (GIT). Found in:

http://www.ncbi.nlm.nih.gov/pubmed/17928638

[2] Konturek, SJ, et al. Role of melatonin in upper gastrointestinal tract. Found In: http://www.ncbi.nlm.nih.gov/pubmed/18212399

[3] Reiter, RJ., et al. Melatonin and its Relation to the Immune System and Inflammation. Found in: http://onlinelibrary.wiley.com/doi/10.1111/j.1749-632.2000.tb05402.x/abstract;jsessionid=CC17DA4C50DE D3932D33CDED42A93472.d03t02?deniedAccessCustomi sedMessage=anduserIsAuthenticated=false

TWELVE

[1] chelators

[2] http://www.tetonsage.com/bacterial-balance/

[3] Hupston, Fleur. Top foods that chelate the body of heavy metals. Found In: http://www.naturalnews.com/038670_heavy_metals_ch elation_foods.html

[4] Bacterial Balance. Found In: http://www.tetonsage.com/bacterial-balance/

Bibliography:

O'shea, Tim. The Post-Anti-biotic Age: Germ Theory. Found in: http://www.whale.to/vaccine/shea1.html

Different theory between western Medicine and Traditional Chinese Medicine in the causes of disease. Found in: http://www.chineseherbal.com.au/western_medicine_tcm.htm

Davis, Charles Patrick. Medical Microbiology. Chapter 6 Normal Flora. Found in: http://www.ncbi.nlm.nih.gov/books/NBK7617/

www.ingramcontent.com/pod-product-compliance
Lightning Source LLC
Chambersburg PA
CBHW071232290326
41931CB00037B/2841